Ketogenic diet cookbook for beginners

Ketogenic diet cookbook: 52 high-fat Desserts Recipes to Lose Weight, Regain Confidence, and Heal Your Body, A Step by Step Guide

(Ingredients & nutritional facts)

By "Wiley Pearson"

©2018

TABLE OF CONTENT

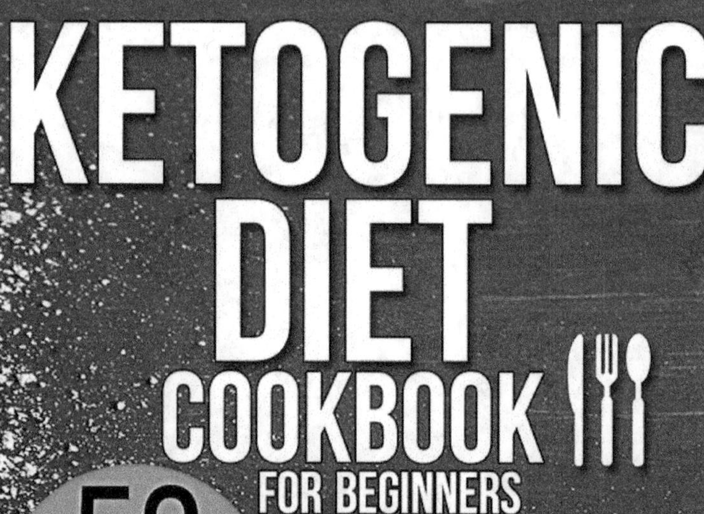

KETOGENIC
DIET
COOKBOOK
FOR BEGINNERS
to Lose Weight Regain Confidence, and
Heal Your Body, A Step by Step Guide
ingredients & nutritional facts
52
HIGH-FAT
DESSERTS RECIPES

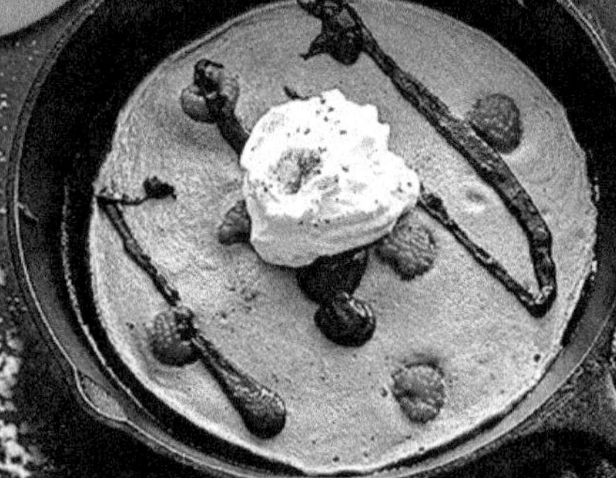

WILEY PEARSON

ABOUT THE AUTHOR

Wiley Pearson is the pen name of the author behind the Ketogenic Diet Book series

A professional chef for over 25 years, Wiley Pearson is a passionate advocate for the Ketogenic diet and the health benefits of a low-carb lifestyle. His areas of expertise include recipe development, holistic health, and medically restricted diets.

He is one of the world's leaders of using dietary change to help balance moods, sharpen brain function and improve mental health. His work focuses on the treatment of depression and anxiety with a combination of diet, lifestyle modification to help people live their healthiest, happiest lives.

Wiley Pearson Spent more than 25 years helping people lose weight, overcome health challenges and reach their ideal health while still enjoying real food and not going hungry

I'm a normal man, having normal life, married with one child and I'm scripting this book due to the fact I need to help human beings as I got assist from near friend that point which surely modified my life.

Want you all the pleasant,

Wiley Pearson

OTHER BOOKS BY <u>THE AUTHOR</u>

<u>Ketogenic Diet</u>

The complete guide to a high-fat diet, free recipes for busy people on the Keto diet, easy meal plans heal your body, and regain your self-confidence

"Your Essential Guide to Keto"

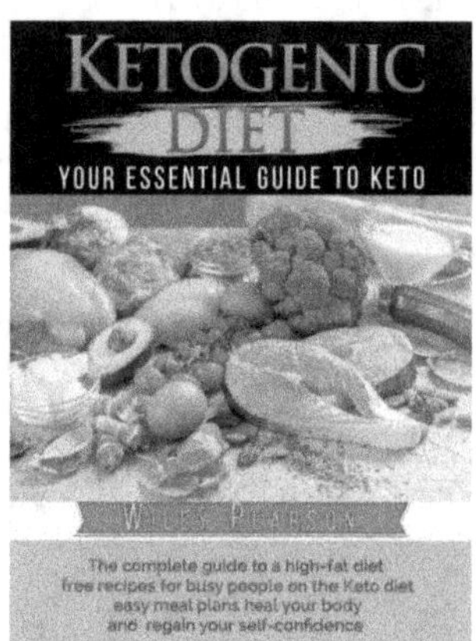

Why I wrote this book?

I wrote this book as I want you to escape the Dieting Trap and Transform Your Life

Have you been spinning your wheels, trying diet after diet, only to lose and regain the same 10, 20, or 30 pounds over and over again? Author Ari Whitten's here to tell you that it's not your fault! The common weight loss strategy of "burn more calories than you take in" will fail 95% of you in the long term, simply because this goes against your body's natural wisdom. So it's time to stop fighting against your biology and start working with your biology. Forever Fat Loss will show you how.

Why you should read this book?

Do you feel that you haven't been honored with the best fat consuming hereditary qualities? Does sustenance appear to go straight to your concern territories like your paunch, bum and thighs?

Do you sense that you've attempted each diet known to man however the weight continues returning?

Imagine a scenario in which I revealed to you that you could get thinner, can rest easy, look better, have more energy, decrease torment, help your sex drive, anticipate infection ... and best of all despite everything you'll have the capacity to in any case eat a portion of the sustenance you desire the most and still experience a slimmer body.

In Ketogenic Diet that is precisely what you'll get

You will find the correct science behind how we put on and get in shape and in addition what completely should be done to assault that tenacious muscle versus fat; that as of recently has been so testing to dispose of. The procedures in this book are so basic, so natural to actualize thus effective... That it will presumably stable so mind boggling when you first read about it.

This weight pulverizing day by day propensities will convey you an aggregate body changeover with no supplements, sweat-soaked exercises or overrated ineffectual weight reduction pills. It will deal with individuals of any weight, anyone shape and anyone write.

Is this book for you?

Getting in shape is similarly as simple as ever on the off chance that you will change some of your day by day propensities, so it is your choice

In this book we will discover how to prepare 52 low carbohydrate delicious desserts within few minutes by using few ingredients and step by step preparation methods

What's in this Cookbook?

52 low carb dessert recipes all using just 5-6 ingredients and 5 net carbs or fewer!

Caloric and macronutrient data– we calculated everything for you so you can track your meals easily.

Low carb and Keto diet basics for beginners and seasoned low carb alike.

Helpful recipe notes and lots of tips for progress and meal tracking

With Ketogenic diet cookbook for beginners, succeeding in your low carb diet has never been easier.

Why   **52**   **Desserts?**
When you started the Keto diet, you probably thought that was the end of dessert. We're here to show you how silly that is! With Ketogenic diet cookbook for beginners, you get 52 mouthwatering recipes that will blow you away each and every time.

Beyond Weight Control

Keto has its origins in treating healthcare conditions such as epilepsy, type 2 diabetes, cardiovascular disease, metabolic syndrome, auto-brewery syndrome and high blood pressure, will take you beyond typical weight control and into a new realm of total body health.

Simple   **and**   **Delicious**
Ketogenic diet cookbook for beginners, delicious, low carb (Keto) dessert recipes that are each made with just 5-6 common ingredients and are 0.5gram up to 5 grams of net carbs! There's nothing better than that.

Low   **Carb**   **Made**   **Easy**
Enjoy chocolate soufflés, brownies, coconut cream pies, Cheesy Hazelnut Morsels and much more every day of the month. Living a low carb lifestyle has never been more enjoyable and sustainable!

Finally, a Diet You Will Enjoy

This Ketogenic cookbook rekindles your love for food, meaning you will look forward to your every meal. When you enjoy what you are eating the results come easy!

Being Low Carb is Easier than Ever!

An average of 3 Net Carbs per Serving
You can count the carbs in each dessert on one hand! Go ahead, have seconds, you'll still be within your daily carb limit.

Only 5-6 Ingredients per Recipe
cutting down the amount of ingredients reduces cost, time, complexity and even the willpower needed to cook. Less is more.

Nutritional Information
Unlike other cookbooks, our recipes include an exact calorie count broken down into fat, carbs and protein to ensure you stay on track for your goals, we calculated each recipe so you don't have to.

Join millions of others across the globe by ditching fad diets and turning to a proven solution which does not sacrifice taste or enjoyment of eating.

Ketogenic Diet life style,

The Ketogenic diet is a high-fat, moderate-protein, low-carbohydrate diet that was utilized before to treat epilepsy in children who did not recuperate well to the accessible epilepsy medicines around then.

This diet style upholds the body to utilize and consume fats as the fundamental wellspring of energy over than utilizing carbohydrates. The body changes the taken carbohydrates in our nourishment into glucose which later is sent all through the body to be used as energy. Shockingly, if your carbohydrates intake is higher than your body needs for the amount of energy you use during a day, the overabundance glucose is changed over fats and stored rather than being burned causing weight gain.

Be that as it may, in the event that you confine the measure of carbohydrates ingested, the liver will start changing over fat into unsaturated fats and ketone bodies. When ketones in the blood dwarf the molecules of glucose, the cells of your body will begin to utilize those ketones as their fundamental wellspring of energy.

How Does The Ketogenic Diet Work?

The Ketogenic diet fills in as it moves the body's metabolism from utilizing glucose as energy to utilize ketones to be the principle wellspring of energy. While it doesn't ensure moment weight reduction, it is a compelling diet framework to help you to accomplish your objectives of living in healthier way and make the most of your life.

In the first place, you will be eating extremely fulfilling and nutritious nourishments that will influence you to encounter fewer desires and to be less eager frequently. The present nutritionists won't disclose to you that great fats cause satiation, not foods grown from the ground. It has been resolved through numerous restorative examinations that protein and fats are the most fulfilling of the three macronutrients you will be worried about when following this new way of life.

Second, eating fats really encourages your body to consume the put away fat with the goal that you can shed pounds in a less demanding way.

Carbohydrates make the body create insulin to move glucose particles into the cells to be utilized for energy. Sadly, almost everybody who is overweight for a drawn out stretch of time will encounter some type of insulin-resistance regardless of whether they have not been analyzed as diabetic.

This implies you will encounter both high and low glucose levels and also more yearnings.

Also, third, you will have the capacity to accomplish more prominent weight loss because of the metabolic preferred standpoint the low-carbohydrates diet underpins.

At the point when your liver separate fats there are constantly a greater number of ketones than your body can really utilize, so the overabundance is discharged through pee

In any case, that loss of potential energy isn't excessively extraordinary so you won't miss it.

Comparison between Ketogenic Diet and 'Traditional' Diets

You may have attempted maybe a couple – or many – of the more traditional diets and had a long time to a couple of months worth of weight reduction yet thought that it was anything but difficult to … suppose, fudge your diet? Furthermore, I imply that actually – fudge can be a major destruction. Am I right?

Presently we can Compare the accompanying two records and perceive how the Ketogenic diet can help you to accomplish your weight loss objectives.

Traditional Diet

- ✓ Restricts fat admission

- ✓ Allows for direct protein admission

- ✓ Increases leafy foods consumption (fruits and vegetables)

- ✓ Follows Food Pyramid rules

- ✓ Restricts caloric admission

- ✓ Doesn't enable changes in accordance with decrease abundance hunger

- ✓ Doesn't mitigate longings

- ✓ May require obtaining extraordinarily bundled dinners relying upon what diet is being taken after

Ketogenic Diet

- ✓ Restricts carbohydrates consumption

- ✓ Allows for direct protein consumption

- ✓ Increases advantageous fat admission

- ✓ Flips the Food Pyramid rules on its head

- ✓ Restricting caloric admission isn't completely vital

- ✓ Allows change in accordance with decrease abundance hunger

- ✓ Alleviates most, if not all, desires

- ✓ Doesn't require uniquely bought sustenance unless you do as such

As should be obvious, the Ketogenic diet is the inverse of any traditional diet you may have attempted. Perhaps that is the reason it works so well.

DELIGHTFUL DESSERTS

MINIATURE CHEESECAKES

Enough to serve 12

Preparation time: 10 minutes   cook time: 35 minutes   total time required for preparation: 50 minutes

In my opinion, cheesecake is the almost-perfect Keto dessert except for its sugar and crust. Here, I make the crust with almond flour and the filling with Stevia instead of cane sugar. When one of those chocolate cravings hits, I like to add chunks of dark chocolate or small pieces of fruit. Play around with your favorite add-ins to the make this dessert recipe your own.

INGREDIENTS:

- ✗ 4 tablespoons butter
- ✗ ½ cup almond flour
- ✗ 2 cups cream cheese, at room temperature
- ✗ ¼ cup Stevia or other sugar substitute
- ✗ 1 Teaspoon pure vanilla extract
- ✗ ½ Teaspoon freshly squeezed lemon juice

Preparation Steps:

1. Preheat the oven to 300°F.

2. In a medium microwaveable bowl, microwave the butter on high for 20 seconds, or until melted. Add the almond flour to the bowl. Mix to combine.

3. In a cupcake pan, divide the almond flour crust evenly among the cups. Press the mixture firmly into the bottom of each. Place the pan in the preheated oven. Bake for 10 minutes. Remove from the oven. Set aside.

4. In a large bowl, mix together the cream cheese, stevia, vanilla, and lemon juice.

5. Top each crust with an equal amount of the cream cheese batter.

6. Return the pan to the oven. Bake for 15 minutes.

7. Increase the heat to 350°F. Bake for 10 minutes more.

8. Remove from the oven. Cool for 5 minutes.

NUTRITIONAL FACTS PER SERVING (1 MINI CHEESECAKE)

- Ratio: 3:1

- Calories: 227

- Total fat: 19.5g

- Total carbohydrates: 13.9g

- Net total carbohydrates: 13.4g

- Fiber: 0.5g

- Protein: 2.9g

CHOCOLATE MUG CAKE

Enough to serve 1

Total time required for preparation: 10 minutes

This is the Keto-version of the now famous chocolate mug cake. Made with Stevia instead of sugar and aided by extra egg, this fluffy, delicious chocolate cake will delight you. Top with whipped cream or serve with fresh berries for an added treat.

INGREDIENTS:

- Cooking spray
- 2 tablespoons cocoa powder
- 2 tablespoons Stevia or other sugar substitute
- Pinch salt
- 1 tablespoon heavy (whipping) cream
- ½ Teaspoon pure vanilla extract
- 1 egg, beaten
- ¼ Teaspoon baking powder

Preparation Steps:

1. Spray the inside of a microwaveable mug with cooking spray.
2. In a medium bowl, mix together the cocoa powder, Stevia, and salt.
3. Add the heavy cream, vanilla, and the beaten egg. Mix to combine. Add the baking powder and mix again.
4. Continue mixing until there are no air bubbles.
5. Transfer the batter to the prepared mug. Microwave on high for 1 minute, 20 seconds.
6. Remove the cake from the microwave. Allow it to settle for 1 minute before inverting onto a plate to serve.

NUTRITIONAL FACTS PER SERVING (1 CAKE)

- Ratio: 3:1

- Calories: 146
- Total fat: 11.3g
- Total carbohydrates: 7.5g
- Net total carbohydrates: 4.3g
- Fiber: 3.2
- Protein: 7.8g

CHOCOLATE PEANUT BUTTER FAT BOMBS

Enough to serve 16

Total time required for preparation: 1¼ hours

When my legendary chocolate cravings hit, I reach for these peanut buttery cups of high-fat bliss. This recipe seamlessly blends coconut oil with peanut butter powder to create a smooth texture. If I only have regular peanut butter on hand, I just decrease the amount of coconut oil by about 1 tablespoon. My favorite way to eat these is to take small bites and let them slowly melt.

INGREDIENTS:

- 4 tablespoons butter

- 4 tablespoons coconut oil

- 4 tablespoons heavy whipping cream

- 2 tablespoons powdered peanut butter, like PB2

- 2 tablespoons unsweetened cocoa powder

- 1 Teaspoon pure vanilla extract

- 1 Teaspoon Stevia, or other sugar substitute

Preparation Steps:

1. To a medium microwaveable bowl, add the butter and coconut oil. Microwave on high in short 10-second intervals until the mixture begins to melt. Once melted, add the heavy cream. Whisk thoroughly to combine.

2. Mix in the powdered peanut butter, cocoa powder, vanilla, and Stevia.

3. Pour the mixture evenly into an ice cube tray. Freeze for at least 1 hour to solidify, preferably overnight.

4. Enjoy within 2 hours.

NUTRITIONAL FACTS PER SERVING (1 BOMB)

- Ratio: 4:1

- Calories: 73
- Total fat: 7.8g
- Total carbohydrates: 1g
- Net total carbohydrates: 0.5g
- Fiber: 0.5g
- Protein: 0.6g

DOUBLE CHOCOLATE BROWNIES

Enough to serve 8

Preparation time: 10 minutes   cook time: 30 minutes   total time required for preparation: 45 minutes

Rich, dark chocolate is the shining star in this double chocolate brownie recipe. Sprinkled with dark chocolate, these gooey, almond flour–based brownies are good to the last crumb. Garnish with a dollop of whipped cream or some sliced berries.

<u>INGREDIENTS:</u>

- ✗ ¼ cup almond flour
- ✗ ½ cup Stevia or other sugar substitute
- ✗ 3 tablespoons cocoa powder
- ✗ ½ Teaspoon baking powder
- ✗ ¼ Teaspoon salt
- ✗ 4 tablespoons butter, melted
- ✗ 3 eggs
- ✗ 1 Teaspoon pure vanilla extract
- ✗ ¼ cup 90 percent dark chocolate, crumbled

<u>Preparation Steps:</u>

1. Preheat the oven to 350°F.

2. In a large bowl, combine the almond flour, stevia, cocoa powder, baking powder, and salt. Whisk to combine.

3. In a medium bowl, whisk together the butter, eggs, and vanilla.

4. Add the butter mixture to the almond flour. Stir to combine.

5. Incorporate the dark chocolate into the batter. Transfer the batter to an 8-inch-square baking pan.

6. Place the pan in the preheated oven. Cook for 30 minutes.

7. Remove the pan from the oven. Cool the brownies for at least 5 minutes before cutting into 8 portions.

<u>NUTRITIONAL FACTS PER SERVING (1 BROWNIE)</u>

- Ratio: 4:1

- Calories: 191

- Total fat: 17.2g

- Total carbohydrates: 5.5g

- Net total carbohydrates: 2.9g

- Fiber: 2.6g

- Protein: 3.2g

PEANUT BUTTER COOKIES

Enough to Make 25

Preparation time: 10 minutes   cook time: 13 minutes   total time required for preparation: 25 minutes

Peanut butter and cream cheese come together to create this unique, chewy cookie. Crunchy on the outside but chewy on the inside, these mimic the traditional peanut butter cookie in many ways. The dough will be very sticky, so wet your hands before forming the cookies.

INGREDIENTS:

- 1 cup sugar-free peanut butter

- ½ cup cream cheese, at room temperature

- 20 drops liquid Stevia or other liquid sugar substitute

- 1 egg

- 1 Teaspoon pure vanilla extract

Preparation Steps:

1. Preheat the oven to 350°F.

2. In a large bowl, combine the peanut butter, cream cheese, Stevia, egg, and vanilla. Mix thoroughly to combine. Divide the dough by heaping tablespoons into 25 equal portions. Form into balls.

3. On parchment-lined baking sheets, arrange the cookie balls at least 1 inch apart.

4. With a fork, flatten each cookie, crisscrossing the imprint with the tines.

5. Place the baking sheets in the oven. Bake for 12 to 13 minutes, or until golden brown.

6. Cool the cookies for 2 to 3 minutes before serving. Store in an airtight container.

NUTRITIONAL FACTS PER SERVING (1 COOKIE)

- Ratio: 3:1

- Calories: 79
- Total fat: 6.9g
- Total carbohydrates: 2.2g
- Net total carbohydrates: 1.6g
- Fiber: 0.6 g
- Protein: 3.1g

CHOCOLATE-COVERED BACON

Enough to serve 4

Preparation time: 15 minutes   cook time: 20 minutes   total time required for preparation: 1½ hours

Chocolate and bacon, two of life's most sinful pleasures, come together in this decadent, savory, and sweet recipe. Skewering the bacon allows the chocolate to adhere well to the meat, though it is not necessary. If you work without the skewers, simply cook the bacon flat in a pan, transfer to parchment paper, and brush on the chocolate.

INGREDIENTS:

- ✗ 8 bacon slices

- ✗ 1½ tablespoons coconut oil

- ✗ 3 tablespoons unsweetened chocolate chips or pieces

- ✗ 1 Teaspoon Stevia or other sugar substitute

Preparation Steps:

1. Preheat the oven to 425°F.

2. Skewer each bacon slice accordion-style.

3. Place on a baking sheet. Put the sheet in the preheated oven. Bake for 15 minutes, until crisp.

4. Remove the bacon from the oven and cool completely.

5. In a medium saucepan over low heat, melt the coconut oil and chocolate. Whisk in the Stevia.

6. Transfer the bacon to a sheet of parchment paper. With a pastry brush, coat one side of each bacon slice with some of the chocolate. Flip. Coat the other side of each piece with the remaining chocolate.

7. Refrigerate for 1 hour before serving.

NUTRITIONAL FACTS PER SERVING (2 CHOCOLATE-COVERED BACON SLICES)

- Ratio: 3:1

- Calories: 214

- Total fat: 12.8g

- Total carbohydrates: 3.2g

- Net total carbohydrates: 1.8g

- Fiber: 1.4g

- Protein: 9.4g

CHOCOLATE COCONUT MILK ICE CREAM

Enough to serve 1

Total time required for preparation: 35 minutes

Ice cream is not very Keto friendly, but when made this unique way with coconut milk you get the same creamy consistency without the added sugar. Enjoy this with unsweetened coconut flakes, cocoa nibs, or shaved dark chocolate. You can make vanilla flavored ice cream by replacing the cocoa powder with 1 Teaspoon of vanilla extract.

INGREDIENTS:

- ½ cup coconut milk

- 1 tablespoon heavy whipping cream

- 1 tablespoon unsweetened cocoa powder

Preparation Steps:

1. In a large bowl, whisk the coconut milk, heavy cream, and cocoa powder for 2 minutes, until it thickens and forms stiff peaks.

2. Transfer the mixture to a freezer safe container. Freeze for 20 to 30 minutes, until set to your desired consistency.

NUTRITIONAL FACTS PER SERVING (1 RECIPE)

- Ratio: 4:1

- Calories: 340

- Total fat: 34.9g

- Total carbohydrates: 10g

- Net total carbohydrates: 5.6g

- Fiber: 4.4g

- Protein: 4.1g

Almond Butter Fat Bombs

Enough to Make: 24

Total time required for preparation: 22 minutes

Ingredients

- 2 1/2 cup almond butter
- 1/2 cup shredded coconut (unsweetened)
- 2 eggs
- 1/2 cup Stevia sweetener
- 1 Tbsp pure vanilla extract

Preparation Steps:

1. Preheat oven to 320 F. Line square baking tray with baking paper.
2. Place all ingredients in a bowl. Knead the mixture by your hands.
3. After the ingredients are mixed, roll into heaped teaspoon sized balls and place into a baking tray.
4. Bake in the oven for 12 minutes or until the tops of the cookies are browning. Let cool on a wire rack. Serve.

Nutrition Facts per serving

- Total Carbohydrates: 5.6g
- Dietary Fiber: 1.8g
- Net Total Carbohydrates: 2.6g
- Protein: 7.3g
- Total Fat: 14.5g
- Calories: 171

Cheesy Hazelnut Morsels

Enough to Make: 16

Total time required for preparation: 15 minutes

Ingredients

- 1/2 cup ground hazelnuts
- 1/4 cup hazelnut butter
- 1 cup cream cheese
- 1/4 cup cocoa powder
- 2 Tbsp Sugar free Hazelnut syrup
- Natural sweetener of your cheese, to taste

Preparation Steps:

1. In a large bowl, place the softened cream cheese (on room temperature) and hazelnut butter. Add in all other ingredients (except the ground hazelnuts).

2. With a wooden spoon to blend the cream cheese, cocoa powder, butter, syrup and sweetener.

3. In a bowl place the ground hazelnuts. Roll the cream cheese mixture into 16 balls. Dip each ball into the ground hazelnuts.

4. Refrigerate for at least 2-3 hours.

Nutrition Facts per serving

- Total Carbohydrates: 3,4g
- Dietary Fiber: 1,4g
- Net Total Carbohydrates: 1,2g
- Protein: 3,2g
- Total Fat: 11,6g
- Calories: 122

Choco Mint Hazelnut Sticks

Enough to Make: 12

Total time required for preparation: 20 minutes

Ingredients

- 4 Tbsp cocoa powder

- 1 cup shredded coconut

- 1 cup hazelnuts

- 1 tsp peppermint extract

- 6 Tbsp coconut oil, melted

- 4 Tbsp almond butter

- 3/4 cup Stevia sweetener (or some other natural sweetener of your choice)

- 1 tsp vanilla extract

- Pinch of salt

Preparation Steps:

1. In a large bowl stir together the coconut oil, cacao powder, almond butter, sweetener, vanilla, peppermint extract and salt. Chop the hazelnuts in a food processor.

2. Heat the mixture slowly on low heat over simmering water (double boiler) for 5 to 10 minutes until all ingredients are combined well.

3. Add hazelnuts and shredded coconut to the melted chocolate mixture and stir together.

4. Pour in a dish lined with parchment and freeze until chocolate is set then cut into sticks.

Nutrition Facts per serving

- Total Carbohydrates: 5,6g

- Dietary Fiber: 2,4g

- Net Total Carbohydrates: 2g

- Protein: 3g

- Total Fat: 17g

- Calories: 174

Chocolate Keto Bomb Cookies

Enough to Make: 10

Total time required for preparation: 10 minutes

Ingredients

- 1 Tbsp cacao powder
- 2 Tbsp chocolate protein powder
- 4 Tbsp coconut milk
- 2 Tbsp coconut flour
- 2 Tbsp coconut, shredded
- 1 Tbsp cacao nibs
- Topping
- 1 tsp coconut oil, softened
- 2/3 cup coconut butter, softened

Preparation Steps:

- In a bowl combine all ingredients (except ingredients for coating). Whisk 2-3 minutes until well combined.
- Spoon out mixture into small molds.
- Place molds in refrigerator for 30 minutes.
- In a meanwhile prepare coating. In a bowl, mix coconut oil with coconut butter. Remove molds from refrigerator and cover with coating
- Place back to refrigerator until coating has hardened, about 1 hour.

Nutrition Facts per serving

- Total Carbohydrates: 2,55g
- Dietary Fiber: 1g
- Net Total Carbohydrates: 0,71g
- Protein: 1g

- Total Fat: 14,47g

- Calories: 138

COCONUT TRUFFLES

Enough to serve 12

Total time required for preparation: 25 minutes

Unsweetened coconut flakes wrap around rich cream cheese for these quick and easy truffles. Extremely simple, these can be frozen and thawed as needed or refrigerated in an airtight container. Experiment by adding spices, like cinnamon, for a twist.

INGREDIENTS:

- 8 ounces (1 package) cream cheese, at room temperature
- ½ cup Stevia or other sugar substitute
- 2 Teaspoons coconut extract
- ½ cup unsweetened shredded coconut

Preparation Steps:

1. In a medium bowl, mix together the cream cheese, stevia, and coconut extract.

2. Scoop into balls, 1 to 2 tablespoons in size. It should yield about 12.

3. Roll the balls in the coconut flakes. Chill the truffles for 15 minutes before serving.

NUTRITIONAL FACTS PER SERVING (1 TRUFFLE)

- Ratio: 4:1
- Calories: 98
- Total fat: 9.3g
- Total carbohydrates: 1.6g
- Net total carbohydrates: 0.9g
- Fiber: 0.7g
- Protein: 1.8g

Chocolate Peanut Butter Balls

Enough to Make: 12

Total time required for preparation: 10 minutes

Ingredients

- 1/2 stick butter, softened
- 1/2 cup natural peanut butter
- 2 Tbsp coconut flour
- 2 Tbsp vanilla whey protein powder
- 1/2 cup broken up sugar free chocolate bars, melted
- 1 tsp organic vanilla extract
- 1 1/2 cup powdered Xylitol (or some other natural sweetener)

Preparation Steps:

1. In a bowl, mix peanut butter and butter. Beat the butter with an electric hand mixer, beat together butter until smooth.

2. Add in vanilla extract and protein powder to peanut butter mixture, and then mix well.

3. Add in powdered Xylitol sweetener and mix well.

4. On a working surface, roll the dough into 24 two-bite sized balls. Place balls on a pan lined with a parchment paper.

5. Sprinkle each ball with chocolate. Refrigerate for at least 2 hours.

Nutrition Facts per serving

- Total Carbohydrates: 5,16g
- Dietary Fiber: 1,02g
- Net Total Carbohydrates: 2,54g
- Protein: 3g
- Total Fat: 12g

Calories: 126

LEMON CHEESECAKE BARS

Enough to serve 8

Preparation time: 10 minutes   cook time: 2 hours   total time required for preparation: 2½ hours

An almond flour base is accented with a creamy lemon topping in this recipe. The sugar-free gelatin and almond flour crust are what make this recipe Keto-friendly. If you have it on hand, dust these bars with powdered Stevia for added garnish.

INGREDIENTS:

- ½ cup butter, melted
- ½ cup almond flour
- 1 cup boiling water
- ⅓ cup sugar-free lemon gelatin mix
- 8 ounces (1 package) cream cheese
- 2 tablespoons freshly squeezed lemon juice

Preparation Steps:

1. Preheat the oven to 350°F.

2. In a medium bowl, mix together the melted butter and the almond flour. Transfer the mixture to an 8-inch-square baking pan. Press the mixture firmly into the bottom to form a crust.

3. Place the pan in the preheated oven. Bake for 10 minutes. Remove from the oven. Set aside to cool.

4. In large bowl, combine the boiling water and gelatin. Stir for about 2 minutes to dissolve.

5. Add the cream cheese and lemon juice. Mix well to combine.

6. Pour the cream cheese mixture over the cooled crust. Refrigerate for at least 2 hours until set, preferably overnight.

7. Cut into 8 bars and serve.

NUTRITIONAL FACTS PER SERVING (1 LEMON BAR)

- Ratio: 4:1
- Calories: 268
- Total fat: 25.2g
- Total carbohydrates: 2.1g
- Net total carbohydrates: 1.3g
- Fiber: 0.8g
- Protein: 6.5g

Choco-Orange Walnut Muffin Bombs

Enough to Make: 18

Total time required for preparation: 20 minutes

Ingredients

- 1 1/2 cup walnuts, chopped
- 4.4 oz dark chocolate, 100% cocoa
- 1 tsp natural orange extract
- 1 tsp fresh orange peel
- 4 Tbsp extra virgin coconut oil
- 15-20 drops of liquid Stevia
- 1 tsp cinnamon

Preparation Steps:

1. In a heated container of water (water bath) melt the chocolate stirring slightly. Add liquid Stevia, coconut oil and cinnamon. Mix well.

2. Add fresh orange peel and natural orange extract. Add chopped walnuts and mix in well.

3. When ready, with teaspoon place the mixture into small paper muffin.

4. Place in the fridge until solid, at least 4-6 hours.

Nutrition Facts per serving

- Total Carbohydrates: 5g
- Dietary Fiber: 1,5g
- Net Total Carbohydrates: 3g
- Protein: 13g
- Total Fat: 13g
- Calories: 131

Cinnamon Storm Fat Bombs

Enough to Make: 12

Total time required for preparation: 1 hour and 30 minutes

Ingredients

- 1 cup coconut milk
- 1 cup almond butter
- 1 tsp pure vanilla extract
- 3/4 tsp cinnamon
- 1/2 tsp nutmeg
- 1 tsp natural sweetener (choose your taste)
- 1 cup coconut shreds

Preparation Steps:

1. In a double boiler over medium heat place all the ingredients (except shredded coconut). Stir all the time to melt and combine well.

2. When ready, remove from the heat. Let cool for 5-6 minutes. Place the bowl in the fridge about 45 minutes until hard.

3. In a bowl put the coconut shreds. Roll the coconut-cinnamon mixture into one inch balls and roll them through the coconut shreds.

4. Place the balls on a serving plate and refrigerate for 2-3 hours.

Nutrition Facts per serving

- Total Carbohydrates: 1,6g
- Dietary Fiber: 0,5g
- Net Total Carbohydrates: 0,2g
- Protein: 1g
- Total Fat: 20g

Calories: 18

ZUCCHINI MUFFINS

Enough to serve 16

Preparation time: 5 minutes   cook time: 20 minutes   total time required for preparation: 30 minutes

This light, easy to make zucchini muffins are handy to have for a quick breakfast. They are excellent paired with Cinnamon Butter and a cup of Buttered Coffee. Refrigerate in an airtight container to preserve the quality.

INGREDIENTS:

- 1 cup grated, drained zucchini
- 1 cup almond flour
- ¼ cup almond butter
- 3 eggs
- 1 tablespoon honey
- 1 Teaspoon pure vanilla extract
- 1 Teaspoon baking powder
- 1 Teaspoon cinnamon

Preparation Steps:

1. Preheat the oven to 350°F.

2. In a large bowl, combine the zucchini, almond flour, almond butter, eggs, honey, vanilla, baking powder, and cinnamon. Mix well.

3. Line a cupcake pan with paper liners. Divide the batter evenly among the paper liners.

4. Place the pan in the preheated oven. Bake for 18 to 20 minutes, or until golden brown.

5. Cool the muffins for 5 minutes before serving.

NUTRITIONAL FACTS PER SERVING (1 MUFFIN)

- Ratio: 3:1
- Calories: 184

- Total fat: 14.9g

- Total carbohydrates: 6.7g

- Net total carbohydrates: 4.9g

- Fiber: 1.8g

- Protein: 4.8g

Keto Orange Fat Bites

Enough to Make: 14

Total time required for preparation: 10 minutes

Ingredients

- 1/2 cup heavy whipping cream
- 1/2 cup cream cheese
- 1/2 cup coconut oil, melted
- 1 tsp pure orange extract
- 10 drops Liquid Stevia (or the natural sweetener of your choice)

Preparation Steps:

1. In an immersion blender place all ingredients. Blend until corporate well.
2. Add in orange extract and liquid Stevia and mix together with a spoon.
3. Spread the batter mixture into a silicone tray, or in paper muffins trays.
4. Refrigerate for 2 hours. Before serving remove from silicone tray and serve. Keep refrigerated.

Nutrition Facts per serving

- Total Carbohydrates: 0,5g
- Dietary Fiber: 0g
- Net Total Carbohydrates: 0,3g
- Protein: 1g
- Total Fat: 14g
- Calories: 127

Cocos Nut Bombs

Enough to Make: 12

Total time required for preparation: 15 minutes

Ingredients

- 1 1/2 cup flaked coconut, unsweetened
- 1 cup coconut oil
- 1 cup extra virgin coconut oil
- 1 tsp cinnamon powder
- 1/8 tsp salt
- 2 Tbsp of powdered Erythritol

Preparation Steps:

1. Preheat the oven 350 F.
2. Arrange evenly the flaked coconut on a rectangular baking tray. Place in the oven and toast for 8 minutes strictly. Let cool 2-3 minutes.
3. Transfer baked coconut into a blender and pulse until get a smooth and runny consistency.
4. Add the softened coconut oil, vanilla, Erythritol, salt and cinnamon. Blend well.
5. Pour the mixture with the tablespoon into ice cube tray to get 12 servings. Refrigerate for at least 2-3 hours.
6. Ready. Serve and enjoy! Keep refrigerated.

Nutrition Facts per serving

- Total Carbohydrates: 1,5g
- Dietary Fiber: 1g
- Net Total Carbohydrates: 0,6g
- Protein: 0,4g
- Total Fat: 13g

Calories: 114

Easy Choco Blueberry Fat Bombs

Enough to Make: 6

Total time required for preparation: 15 minutes

Ingredients

- 5 Tbsp butter
- 3 Tbsp coconut oil
- 2 Tbsp sugar-free Blueberry syrup
- 2 Tbsp cocoa powder

Preparation Steps:

1. In a sauce pan add all ingredients and cook over low heat until chocolate sauce texture.
2. Pour into mold and freeze for at least 3 hours.
3. Before serving unmold and enjoy.

Nutrition Facts per serving

- Total Carbohydrates: 1g
- Dietary Fiber: 0,6g
- Net Total Carbohydrates: 0,05
- Protein: 0,5g
- Total Fat: 17g
- Calories: 148

Easy Cream Cheese Jello Balls

Enough to Serve: 8

Total time required for preparation: 10 minutes

Ingredients

- 1 cup cream cheese
- 1/4 cup coconut butter
- 1 package of sugar free jello

Preparation Steps:

1. In a small bowl put the jello powder.
2. In a separate bowl, mix together cream cheese and coconut butter.
3. Take a teaspoon of batter, roll into a ball in your hands and then roll in the jello powder. Make 16 balls.
4. Cover with plastic wrap and place in the fridge.

Nutrition Facts per serving

- Total Carbohydrates: 1,20g
- Dietary Fiber: 0g
- Net Total Carbohydrates: 1g
- Protein: 2g
- Total Fat: 16g
- Calories: 150g

Gingery Coconut Fat Bomb

Enough to Serve: 10

Total time required for preparation: 5 minutes

Ingredients

- 1 tsp dried (powdered) ginger
- 0.8 oz shredded coconut (unsweetened)
- 1/3 cup coconut oil, softened
- 1/3 cup coconut butter, softened
- 1 tsp granulated sweetener of choice, to taste

Preparation Steps:

1. In a deep bowl, mix shredded coconut, coconut oil, coconut butter, sweetener and dried powdered ginger.

2. Pour the ginger mixture into ice block trays and refrigerate for 1 hour to solidify.

Nutrition Facts per serving

- Total Carbohydrates: 2,5g
- Dietary Fiber: 0,25g
- Net Total Carbohydrates: 0,3g
- Protein:
- Total Fat: 14,5g
- Calories: 134

Homemade Keto Almond Butter

Enough to Serve: 14

Total time required for preparation: 40 minutes

Ingredients

- 3 cups almonds (Without any added salt)
- 1 tsp Himalayan salt
- 1 tsp cinnamon
- 1 vanilla pod or bean, halved and seeds removed
- 2 Tbsp Stevia powder or Erythritol sweetener

Preparation Steps:

1. Preheat oven to 360F degrees. Place almonds in a baking pan and bake for 10-12 minutes. Stir occasionally to not burn.

2. Transfer the almonds in a food processor and add remaining ingredients.

3. Process for 15 minutes above. This process takes a time so, you have to be patient. Pour the almond butter to a glass container and store in the refrigerator.

Nutrition Facts per serving

- Total Carbohydrates: 5,5g
- Dietary Fiber: 2,8g
- Net Total Carbohydrates: 1.3g
- Protein: 5g
- Total Fat: 13,5g
- Calories: 153g

Keto Almond Cookies Bombs

Enough to Make: 16

Total time required for preparation: 25 minutes

Ingredients

- 1 cup almonds, chopped
- 1 cup butter, softened
- 2 1/4 cups almond flour
- 1 1/4 cup cocoa powder
- 3 1/2 Tbsp coconut flour
- 2 eggs
- 3/4 cup Stevia powder
- 2 tsp vanilla extract
- 1/2 tsp baking soda
- 1/4 tsp sea salt

Preparation Steps:

1. Preheat oven to 340F degrees.

2. In a bowl, whisk butter and sweetener. Add the eggs, coconut oil and vanilla extract.

3. In a separate bowl, mix together the baking soda, almond flour, coconut flour, cocoa powder and salt.

4. Combine the eggs mixture to the flour mixture. Pour dough in a greased baking pan. Sprinkle dough with chopped almond over top.

5. Bake for 15-18 minutes. Let cool and cut into chunks. Serve.

Nutrition Facts per serving

- Total Carbohydrates: 3,35g
- Dietary Fiber: 1g

- Net Total Carbohydrates: 0,5g

- Protein: 2,9g

- Total Fat: 17g

- Calories: 171

Keto Hazelnuts Fat Bomb Squares

Enough to Make: 6

Total time required for preparation: 15 minutes

Ingredients

- 1/2 cup hazelnuts, chopped

- 1 cup whipped cream

- 1/4 cup cocoa butter

- 2 Tbs cocoa powder, unsweetened

- 2 Tbs Stevia sweeteners

- Crushed walnuts (optional extra)

Preparation Steps:

1. In a bowl, melt cocoa butter at room temperature.

2. When ready, add in cocoa powder, Stevia powder and mix well until all ingredients are well blended. Add in chopped hazelnuts and stir well.

3. Finally, add whipping cream and mix well.

4. Pour the hazelnut mixture in squared molds and let cool (Ice trays work just fine)

5. Refrigerate for 1 - 2 hours. Dress with crushed walnuts if so desired Serve.

Nutrition Facts per serving

- Total Carbohydrates: 3,8g

- Dietary Fiber: 1,3g

- Net Total Carbohydrates: 0,5g

- Protein: 2g

- Total Fat: 16,5g

- Calories: 160

Keto Lime Fat Bombs

Enough to Make: 16

Total time required for preparation: 10 minutes

Ingredients

- Fresh lime zest from 2 organic limes
- 1 cup extra virgin coconut oil, softened
- 3/4 cup coconut butter, softened
- 20 drops Erythritol extract (or some other natural sweetener of your choice)
- Pinch of salt

Preparation Steps:

1. Soft the coconut butter and coconut oil on room temperature.
2. Zest the organic limes.
3. In a bowl mix all the ingredients in a bowl and stir well. Make sure that lime zest and Erythritol extract are distributed evenly.
4. Prepare 16 mini muffin cups.
5. Refrigerate for 2 hours. Ready. Keep refrigerated.

Nutrition Facts per serving

- Total Carbohydrates: 0,9g
- Dietary Fiber: 0,3g
- Net Total Carbohydrates: 0,15g
- Protein: 0,2g
- Total Fat: 12,5g
- Calories: 109

Lemon Coconut Fat Bombs

 Enough to Serve: 12

Total time required for preparation: 15 minutes

Ingredients

- 1/4 cup shredded coconut, unsweetened,
- 1 cup cream cheese
- 1 Tbsp pure lemon extract
- Natural sweetener of your choice, to taste
- 1/4 cup butter

Preparation Steps:

1. In a bowl, combine cream cheese, natural sweetener and lemon extract. Blend all ingredients together well with mixing spoon. Place bowl in refrigerator for 15-20 minutes.

2. In a bowl place unsweetened shredded coconut. Roll lemon batter into 16 equal balls.

3. Dip each ball into coconut and place on a serving pan. Refrigerate for 3-4 hours at least. Serve.

Nutrition Facts per serving

- Total Carbohydrates: 1g
- Dietary Fiber: 0,2g
- Net Total Carbohydrates: 0,8g
- Protein: 1,3g
- Total Fat: 12g
- Calories: 106

Lemony Cream Cheese Bombshells

Enough to Serve: 12

Total time required for preparation: 2 hours

Ingredients

- 1/2 cup butter, unsalted and softened
- 1 cup cream cheese, softened
- 1/2 tsp pure lemon extract
- 3/4 cup granular Stevia

Preparation Steps:

1. Place all ingredients in a deep bowl. Beat the mixture with an electric mixer several minutes, until soft.

2. When ready, place cream cheese mixture by teaspoon size, one by one onto a wax paper-lined sheet.

3. Freeze until firm, at least 2 hours. Remove to freezer and serve frozen.

Nutrition Facts per serving

- Total Carbohydrates: 0,8g
- Dietary Fiber: 0g
- Net Total Carbohydrates: 0,7g
- Protein: 1,3g
- Total Fat: 14.5g
- Calories: 134

Heavenly Lemon Quads with Coconut Cream

Enough to Serve: 8

Total time required for preparation: 1 hour and 5 minutes

<u>Ingredients</u>

<u>For Base</u>

- 3/4 cup coconut flakes
- 2 Tbsp coconut oil
- 1 Tbsp ground almonds

<u>For Cream</u>

- 5 eggs
- 1/2 lemon juice
- 1 Tbsp coconut flour
- 1/2 cup Stevia sweetener

<u>Preparation Steps:</u>

<u>For Base</u>

1. Preheat oven to 360F.
2. In a bowl put all base ingredients and with clean hands mix everything well until soft.
3. With coconut oil grease a rectangle oven dish. Pour dough in a baking pan. Bake for 15 minutes until golden brown. Set aside to cool.

<u>For Cream</u>

1. In a bowl or blender, whisk together: eggs, lemon juice, coconut flour and sweetener. Pour over the baked caked evenly.
2. Put pan in the oven and bake 20 minutes more.

3. When ready refrigerate for at least 6 hours. Cut in cubes and serve.

Nutrition Facts per serving

- Total Carbohydrates: 4g

- Dietary Fiber: 2,25g

- Net Total Carbohydrates: 1,4g

- Protein: 5g

- Total Fat: 15g

- Calories: 129

Macadamia Cacao Fat Bombs

Enough to Serve: 24

Total time required for preparation: 6 hours

Ingredients

- 1 cup macadamia nuts, chopped
- 1/2 cup cacao powder
- 2 cups almond flour
- 1/2 cup ground flax
- 3 Tbsp coconut oil (melted)
- 1/3 cup Stevia or natural sweetener of your choice
- 1/3 cup water
- 1/2 tsp pure vanilla extract

Preparation Steps:

1. In a bowl, mix almond flour and flax and cacao powder. Stir in oil, water, sweetener and vanilla. When it is well mixed, stir in chopped hazelnuts.

2. Form the mixture into balls, press flat with palms and place on dehydrator screens.

3. Dehydrate 1 hour at 145, then reduce to 116 and dehydrate for at least 5 hours or until desired dryness is achieved.

Nutrition Facts per serving

- Total Carbohydrates: 7g
- Dietary Fiber: 3g
- Net Total Carbohydrates: 3,4
- Protein: 3,5g
- Total Fat: 13g
- Calories: 143

Minty Keto Galettes

Enough to Serve: 18

Total time required for preparation: 20 minutes

Ingredients

- 3 cup coconut butter, melted
- 1 cup coconut, shredded
- 3 Tbsp coconut oil melted
- 3/4 tsp pure peppermint extract
- 2 Tbsp cacao powder

Preparation Steps:

1. In a bowl, mix together, 1 tablespoon of coconut oil and peppermint extract, shredded coconut and melted coconut butter.

2. Pour coconut butter mixture into mini muffin tins by filling half way. Put in refrigerator for about 20 minutes.

3. In a separate bowl mix together 2 tablespoons coconut oil and cacao powder.

4. After 20 minutes remove muffin tin from refrigerator and pour each with cacao mixture.

5. Return to refrigerator for 3-4 hours.

Nutrition Facts (per serving)

- Total Carbohydrates: 0,5g
- Dietary Fiber: 0,3g
- Net Total Carbohydrates: 0,1g
- Protein: 0,25g
- Total Fat: 11g
- Calories: 93

Peanut Butter Cake with Chocolate Sauce

Enough to Serve: 12

Total time required for preparation: 5 minutes

Ingredients

- 1 cup peanut butter
- 1/4 cup almond milk, unsweetened
- 1 cup coconut oil
- 2 tsp liquid Stevia sweetener to taste
- Topping: Chocolate Sauce
- 2 Tbsp coconut oil, melted
- 4 Tbsp cocoa powder, unsweetened
- 2 Tbsp Stevia sweetener

Preparation Steps:

1. In a microwave bowl mix coconut oil and peanut butter; melt in a microwave for 1-2 minutes.

2. Add this mixture to your blender; add in the rest of the ingredients and blend well until combined.

3. Pour the peanut mixture into a parchment lined loaf pan or platter.

4. Refrigerate for about 3 hours; the longer, the better.

5. In a bowl, whisk all topping ingredients together. Pour over the peanut candy after it's been set. Cut into cubes and serve.

Nutrition Facts per serving

- Total Carbohydrates: 5,8g
- Dietary Fiber: 2g
- Net Total Carbohydrates: 2,4g

- Protein: 6g

- Total Fat: 27g

- Calories: 273

Peppermint Fat Bombs

Enough to Serve: 25

Total time required for preparation: 10 minutes

Ingredients

- ✘ 1 1/4 cup seed butter
- ✘ 1 tsp peppermint extract
- ✘ 1 1/2 cups coconut oil
- ✘ 1/2 cup sweetener (liquid or granulated)
- ✘ 2 tsp organic vanilla extract
- ✘ 1/4 tsp salt

Preparation Steps:

1. In a small saucepan melt the coconut oil.

2. In a blender add all remaining ingredients and add melted coconut oil. Blend it until smooth well.

3. With the teaspoon grab the coconut mixture and make the 25 coconut balls.

4. Place the balls into a baking sheet and freeze until solid. Keep refrigerated.

Nutrition Facts per serving

- Total Carbohydrates: 8g
- Dietary Fiber: 1.2g
- Net Total Carbohydrates: 0,25g
- Protein: 2.25g
- Total Fat: 19g
- Calories: 202

Pistachio Masala Fat Bombs

Enough to Serve: 32

Total time required for preparation: 15 minutes

Ingredients

- 1 cup almond butter, melted
- 1/4 cup ghee
- 1 cup coconut oil
- 1/2 cup cocoa butter
- 1/4 cup pistachio nuts
- 1 Tbs coconut milk
- 1 Tbsp pure vanilla extract
- 2 tsp Masala chai (a flavored tea beverage made by brewing black tea with a mixture of aromatic Indian spices and herbs)

Preparation Steps:

1. In a small saucepan melt the cocoa butter over LOW heat.

2. In a large bowl add all ingredients (except the cocoa butter and pistachios).

3. Use a hand mixer and mix well (on HIGH) all ingredients until the mixture combine evenly. Add in the melted butter and continue to blend for 1-2 minutes more.

4. Transfer the mixture to greased and paper lined pan. Sprinkle with chopped pistachios and refrigerate for at least 5 hours.

Nutrition Facts per serving

- Total Carbohydrates: 0,4g
- Dietary Fiber: 0,1g
- Net Total Carbohydrates: 0,1g
- Protein: 0,27 g

- Total Fat: 17g

- Calories: 147

Raspberry Heaven Fat Bombs

Enough to Serve: 18

Total time required for preparation: 15 minutes

Ingredients

- 3 Tbsp heavy cream
- 1/4 cup coconut oil, melted
- 8 oz cream cheese, softened
- 1/4 cup coconut oil, melted
- 3 tsp raspberry extract
- 1/2 cup powdered Erythritol
- Pinch salt
- Few drops of natural red food coloring

Preparation Steps:

1. Prepare the parchment lined baking sheet.
2. In a bowl, with the hand mixer, blend the cream cheese and sweetener together.
3. Add the raspberry extract, natural food coloring cream, salt and raspberry extract and continue to blend.
4. Add in the coconut oil and continue to blend until it's smooth and creamy.
5. Refrigerate this mixture for 1 hour.
6. When ready, make 48 small balls from batter and place into a prepared parchment lined baking sheet. Place it in a freezer for 2 hours.

Nutrition Facts per serving

- Total Carbohydrates: 0,6g
- Dietary Fiber: 0g
- Net Total Carbohydrates: 0.4g

- Protein: 0.77g

- Total Fat: 12g

- Calories: 101

Simple Coconut Fat Bombs

Enough to Serve: 10

Total time required for preparation: 5 minutes

Ingredients

- 1 Tbsp shredded coconut
- 1/3 cup coconut oil, melted
- 1/3 cup coconut butter, softened
- 1 tsp granulated sweetener of choice, to taste

Preparation Steps:

1. Prepare the ice cube trays.
2. Mix all the ingredients in a deep bowl until your natural sweetener is dissolved.
3. Pour batter into ice cube trays.
4. Place in refrigerator for 30 minutes.

Nutrition Facts per serving

- Total Carbohydrates: 2,4g
- Dietary Fiber: 0,1g
- Net Total Carbohydrates: 0,3g
- Protein: 0,2g
- Total Fat: 14g
- Calories: 129

Slow Cooker Pecan Nuts Fat Bomb

Enough to Serve: 8

Total time required for preparation: 2 hours and 15 minutes

Ingredients

- 2 cups Pecans nuts, halves
- 4 Tbsp almond butter
- 1 cup Stevia or any other natural sweetener
- 1/4 tsp ground ginger
- 1/4 tsp ground allspice
- 1 1/2 tsp ground cinnamon

Preparation Steps:

1. In a 4-quart Slow Cooker stir the Pecans nuts halves and almond butter until combined.
2. Add Stevia or any natural sweetener of your choice and stir well.
3. Transfer to a bowl, combine spices and sprinkle over nuts.
4. Cover and cook on HIGH for 15 minutes.
5. Turns to low and cook uncovered for about 2 hours or until the nuts are a little crispy.

Nutrition Facts per serving

- Total Carbohydrates: 3,6g
- Dietary Fiber: 2,3g
- Net Total Carbohydrates: 0,88g
- Protein: 2,9g
- Total Fat: 14g
- Calories: 140

Strawberry Fat Bomb Cream-cakes

Enough to Serve: 12

Total time required for preparation: 1 hour and 10 minutes

Ingredients

- 5 strawberries
- 1/2 cup heavy cream
- 5 Tbsp butter
- 5 Tbsp coconut oil
- 3 Tbsp Trivia (or any favorite sweetener)
- 1 peace dark 100%, sugar free chocolate

Preparation Steps:

1. In a bowl, mix heavy cream and the strawberries.

2. With a help of an immersion blender, blend together heavy cream and strawberries.

3. In a separate bowl, add granulated sweetener and the butter; melt butter mixture in the microwave about 30 seconds.

4. Add the butter mixture to a heavy cream and strawberries and blend well.

5. Spoon mixture into your favorite molds. Freeze at least 30 minutes; the longer, the better.

6. Remove mixture from the mold, place on wax paper and melt one piece sugar free chocolate.

7. Pour melted chocolate over the cream and return to freezer for another 30 minutes.

Nutrition Facts per serving

- Total Carbohydrates: 0,6g
- Dietary Fiber: 0,08g
- Net Total Carbohydrates: 0,2g

- Protein: 0,3gr

- Total Fat: 16g

- Calories: 138

Strawberry Fat Bombs Muffins

Enough to Serve: 10

Total time required for preparation: 10 minutes

Ingredients

- 3/4 cup cream cheese, softened

- 1/4 cup butter, softened

- 1/2 cup strawberries, fresh or frozen

- 1 Tbsp pure vanilla extract

- 10–15 drops liquid Stevia

Preparation Steps:

1. In a mixing bowl, place the butter and the cream cheese and eave at room temperature (about 45min) until softened. Do not microwave the butter!

2. In a separate bowl place the strawberries and mash using a fork.

3. Add the liquid Stevia and vanilla extract and mix well. Add the strawberries to the bowl with softened butter and cream cheese. Whisk until all ingredients are well combined.

4. Pour the strawberry mixture into muffin silicon molds. Place in the freezer for about 3-4 hours.

5. Before serving, unmold the strawberry muffins and place on a serving dish. Keep refrigerated.

Nutrition Facts per serving

- Total Carbohydrates: 1,5g

- Dietary Fiber: 0,2g

- Net Total Carbohydrates: 1,1g

- Protein: 1,15g

- Total Fat: 11g

- Calories: 107

Walnuts Choco Fat Bombs

Enough to Serve: 10

Total time required for preparation: 10 minutes

Ingredients

- 1/3 cup heavy cream
- 1/2 cup cocoa butter
- 1/2 cup pecans, roughly chopped
- 1/2 cup coconut oil
- 4 Tbsp cocoa powder, unsweetened
- 4 Tbsp Swerve, Stevia or Erythritol sweetener

Preparation Steps:

1. In a microwave dish, place cocoa butter and coconut oil together. Use the defrost setting on your microwave and melt in microwave stove for 10-15 seconds.

2. Add in cocoa powder and whisk well. Pour mixture into a blender with sweetener and cream and blend for 3-4 minutes.

3. Place silicone molds onto a sheet pan and fill halfway with walnuts.

4. Pour the mixture with walnuts and place in refrigerator for 6 hours.

Nutrition Facts per serving

- Total Carbohydrates: 2,23g
- Dietary Fiber: 1,25g
- Net Carbs:0,25g
- Protein: 1g
- Total Fat: 29g
- Calories: 150

Almond Butter Cake with Choco Sauce

Enough to Serve: 12

Total time required for preparation: 5 minutes

Ingredients

- 1 cup almond butter or soaked almonds
- 1/4 cup almond milk, unsweetened
- 1 cup coconut oil
- 2 tsp liquid Stevia sweetener to taste
- Topping: Chocolate Sauce
- 4 Tbsp cocoa powder, unsweetened
- 2 Tbsp almond butter
- 2 Tbsp Stevia sweetener

Preparation Steps:

1. Melt the coconut oil in room temperature.
2. Add all ingredients in a bowl and blend well until combined.
3. Pour the almond butter mixture into a parchment lined platter.
4. Place in refrigerator for 3 hours.
5. In a bowl, whisk all topping ingredients together. Pour over the almond cake after it's been set. Cut into cubes and serve.

Nutrition Facts per serving

- Total Carbohydrates: 9,8g
- Dietary Fiber: 2g
- Net Carbs:2,4g
- Protein: 5,8g
- Total Fat: 23,3g

Calories: 273

Butter Pecan Fat Bombs

Enough to Serve: 2

Ingredients

- ✗ 8 pecan halves

- ✗ 1 Tbs unsalted butter, softened

- ✗ 2 oz Neufchatel cheese

- ✗ 1 tsp orange zest, finely grated

- ✗ Pinch of sea salt

Preparation Steps:

1. Toast the pecans at 350 degrees Fahrenheit for 5-10 minutes, check often to prevent burning.

2. Mix the butter, Neufchatel cheese, and orange zest until smooth and creamy.

3. Spread the butter mixture between the cooled pecan halves and sandwich together.

4. Sprinkle with sea salt

Nutrition Facts per serving

- Total Carbohydrates: 3,31g

- Dietary Fiber: 1,5g

- Net Total Carbohydrates: 1,4g

- Protein: 3g

- Total Fat: 26g

- Calories: 243

IMPORTANT INGREDIENT TIP:

Pecans contain more than 19 vitamins and minerals and are also rich in age defying antioxidants. They're rich in fiber which boosts the health of your heart and Phenol-derivatives antioxidants that help to prevent coronary artery disease.

BLUEBERRY CREAM CHEESE BITES

Enough to serve 16

Total time required for preparation: 1¼ hours

Almost like cheesecake, these Blueberry Cream Cheese Bites are quite the treat. Sweetened naturally by the berries, this minimal ingredient recipe is perfect to keep in the freezer for a sweet snack. Try these with blackberries or raspberries, as well.

INGREDIENTS:

- 4 tablespoons butter
- ¼ cup cream cheese
- 4 tablespoons coconut oil
- 4 tablespoons heavy whipping cream
- ¼ cup blueberries, finely chopped
- 1 Teaspoon pure vanilla extract

Preparation Steps:

1. To a medium microwaveable bowl, add the butter, cream cheese, and coconut oil. Microwave on high in short 10-second intervals until the mixture begins to melt. Once melted, add the heavy cream and blueberries.

2. Transfer the mixture to a blender. Pulse to blend in the blueberries.

3. Add the vanilla and pulse to combine.

4. Pour the mixture evenly into an ice cube tray. Freeze for at least 1 hour to solidify, preferably overnight.

5. Treat yourself within 2 hours.

NUTRITIONAL FACTS PER SERVING (1 BITE)

- Ratio: 4:1
- Calories: 82
- Total fat: 8.9g
- Total carbohydrates: 0.6g

- Net total carbohydrates: 0.6g

- Fiber: 0g

- Protein: 0.4g

Choco Almond Fat Bombs

Enough to Serve: 24

Total time required for preparation: 10 minutes

Ingredients

- 3 Tbsp cocoa powder, unsweetened
- 1 cup almond butter
- 1 cup organic coconut oil
- 3-4 Tbsp sweetener to taste
- Splash of almond extract (optional)

Preparation Steps:

1. In a saucepan over medium heat, melt coconut oil and almond butter. Stir in cocoa powder and sweetener of your choice. Remove from heat and add almond extract.

2. Pour almond mixture into silicone candy molds. Freeze or refrigerated until set.

3. Before using remove from molds and store in a fridge in an air tight container.

Nutrition Facts per serving

- Total Carbohydrates: 0,4g
- Dietary Fiber: 1,22g
- Net Total Carbohydrates: 0g
- Protein: 0,5g
- Total Fat: 9,6g
- Calories: 75

COCONUT LEMON FAT BOMBS

Enough to serve 16

Total time required for preparation: 1¼ hours

Fat bombs are the perfect dessert to help you reach your fat macronutrient goal for the day. These Coconut Lemon Fat Bombs get a punch from lemon extract to help the lemon flavor shine through. Add unsweetened coconut flakes for added texture.

INGREDIENTS:

- 2 ounces cream cheese
- 4 tablespoons butter
- 4 tablespoons coconut oil
- 4 tablespoons heavy (whipping) cream
- 2 tablespoons freshly squeezed lemon juice
- 1 Teaspoon lemon extract
- 1 Teaspoon Stevia or other sugar substitute

Preparation Steps:

1. To a medium microwaveable bowl, add the cream cheese, butter, and coconut oil. Microwave on high in short 10-second intervals until the mixture begins to melt. Once melted, add the heavy cream. Whisk thoroughly to combine.

2. Mix in the lemon juice, lemon extract, and Stevia.

3. Pour the mixture evenly into an ice cube tray. Freeze for at least 1 hour to solidify, preferably overnight.

4. Enjoy within 2 hours.

NUTRITIONAL FACTS PER SERVING (1 BOMB)

- Ratio: 4:1
- Calories: 81
- Total fat: 8.9g

- Total carbohydrates: 0.4g

- Net total carbohydrates: 0.4g

- Fiber: 0.4g

- Protein: 0.4g

IMPORTANT INGREDIENT TIP:

If lemon extract and lemon juice are not lemony enough for you, grate some lemon rind and add 1 Teaspoon to the mixture. Meyer lemons have an intense flavor, so use them when possible.

Chocolate-Coconut Layered Cups

Enough to Serve: 10

Ingredients

Bottom Layer:

- 1/2 cup coconut butter
- 1/2 cup coconut oil
- 1/2 cup unsweetened, shredded coconut
- 3 Tbsp powdered sweetener such as Splenda or Trivia

Top Layer:

- 1/2 cup cocoa butter
- 1 oz unsweetened chocolate
- 1/4 cup powdered sweetener such as Splenda or Trivia
- 1/4 cup cocoa powder
- 1/2 tsp vanilla extract

Preparation Steps:

1. Prepare a mini-muffin pan with 20 mini paper liners.

2. For the bottom layer:

3. Combine coconut butter and coconut oil in a small saucepan over low heat. Stir until smooth and melted then add the shredded coconut and powdered sweetener until combined.

4. Divide the mixture among prepared mini muffin cups and freeze until firm, about 30 minutes.

5. For the top layer:

6. Combine cocoa butter and unsweetened chocolate together in double boiler or a bowl set over a pan of simmering water. Stir until melted.

7. Stir in the powdered sweetener, then the cocoa powder and mix until smooth.

8. Remove from heat and stir in the vanilla extract.

9. Spoon chocolate topping over chilled coconut candies and let set, about 15 minutes.

Nutrition Facts per serving

- Total Carbohydrates: 2,7g

- Dietary Fiber: 1,5g

- Net Total Carbohydrates: 0,35g

- Protein: 1g

- Total Fat: 27,5g

- Calories: 247

IMPORTANT INGREDIENT TIP:

Chocolate contains antioxidants known as Polyphenols. Polyphenols play an important role in the prevention of degenerative diseases such as cancer and cardiovascular diseases.

Chocolate-Walnut Fat Bombs

Enough to Serve: 14

Ingredients

- 1/2 cup coconut oil
- 1 oz cocoa powder
- 1 Tbs sugar substitute
- 1 oz walnut pieces
- 1 Tbs tahini paste
- Walnut halves for topping the fat bombs

Preparation Steps:

1. Warm the coconut oil in the microwave until melted.
2. Add the remaining ingredients and stir until well combined.
3. Pour into silicone ice cube trays and refrigerate until almost set.
4. Once almost set, add walnut halves to the top of each fat bomb.
5. Return to fridge until firm.
6. Remove from silicone molds and store in an airtight container in the fridge for up to a week.

Nutrition Facts per serving

- Total Carbohydrates: 2,5g
- Dietary Fiber:1g
- Net Total Carbohydrates: 1g
- Protein: 0,7g
- Total Fat: 10g
- Calories: 88,5

Walnuts have been touted as one of the world's most healthiest foods. Research shows that walnut consumption may support brain health and improve cell function. They contain a good amount of healthy omega-3 fats and are delicious to boot!

Walnuts have been touted as one of the world's most healthiest foods. Research shows that walnut consumption may support brain health and improve cell function. They contain a good amount of healthy omega-3 fats and are delicious to boot!

Cinnamon Bun Fat Bomb Balls

Enough to Serve: 10

Total time required for preparation: 15 minutes

Ingredients

- 1 cup coconut butter
- 1 cup full fat coconut milk
- 1 cup unsweetened coconut shreds
- 1 tsp vanilla extract
- 1/2 tsp cinnamon
- 1/2 tsp nutmeg
- 1 tsp sugar substitute such as Splenda

Preparation Steps:

1. Combine all ingredients except the shredded coconut together in double boiler or a bowl set over a pan of simmering water. Stir until everything is melted and combined.

2. Remove bowl from heat and place in the fridge until the mixture has firmed up and can be rolled into balls.

3. Form the mixture into 1" balls, a small cookie scoop is helpful for doing this.

4. Roll each ball in the shredded coconut until well coated.

5. Serve and Store in the fridge.

Nutrition Facts per serving

- Total Carbohydrates: 2g
- Dietary Fiber: 1g
- Net Total Carbohydrates: 0,6g
- Protein: 0,7g

IMPORTANT INGREDIENT TIP:

Cinnamon is not only delicious, but it's one of the healthiest spices on the planet! It can help to lower blood sugar levels and reduce heart disease risk factors. It's also loaded with powerful antioxidants.

Coconut and Matcha Fat Bomb Balls

Enough to Serve: 32

Ingredients

For the truffles:

- 1 cup firm coconut oil (refrigerate if necessary)
- 1 cup coconut butter
- 1/2 cup full fat coconut milk, refrigerated overnight
- 1/2 tsp matcha green tea powder
- 1/4 tsp cinnamon
- 1/4 tsp sea salt
- 1 tsp pure vanilla extract

For the truffle coating:

- 1 cup finely shredded, unsweetened coconut
- 1 Tbs matcha green tea powder

Preparation Steps:

1. Combine all of the truffle ingredients in a medium sized mixing bowl. Note that it's very important for your coconut oil be firm so send it to the fridge for a little bit if you have to. Same goes for the coconut milk - the thick cream will rise to the top and coconut water will sink to the bottom. While it's not mandatory that you use only the cream part, your milk should be very firm when you use it so make sure that you cool the can overnight.

2. Mix on high speed with a hand mixer, until light and fluffy, then place in the refrigerator to firm up for about an hour.

3. While the truffle mixture is firming up, combine the shredded coconut and matcha powder together in a large, shallow dish. Set aside.

4. With the help of a small cookie scoop form the cold truffle mixture into 32 little balls, roughly the size of a ping pong ball.

5. Roll the balls quickly between the palms of your hands to shape them into perfect little spheres, then drop each ball into the coconut/matcha mixture and roll them until completely coated.

6. Transfer your finished fat bomb balls to an airtight container and keep refrigerated for up to 2 weeks.

7. These can be eaten straight out of the fridge but taste best when you let them sit at room temperature for 10 to 15 minutes before to eat them.

<u>Nutrition Facts per serving</u>

- Total Carbohydrates: 0,6g

- Dietary Fiber: 0,3g

- Net Total Carbohydrates: 0,2g

- Protein: 0,2g

- Total Fat: 14g

- Calories: 123

Coconut-Raspberry Fat Bombs

Enough to Serve: 12

Ingredients

- 1/2 cup coconut butter
- 1/2 cup coconut oil
- 1/2 cup freeze dried raspberries
- 1/2 cup unsweetened shredded coconut
- 1/4 powdered sugar substitute such as Swerve or Trivia

Preparation Steps:

1. Line an 8"x8" pan with parchment paper.
2. In a food processor, coffee grinder, or blender, pulse the dried raspberries into a fine powder.
3. In a saucepan over medium heat, combine the coconut butter, coconut oil, coconut, and sweetener. Stir until melted and well combined.
4. Remove pan from heat and stir in raspberry powder.
5. Pour mixture into pan and refrigerate or freeze for several hours, or overnight.
6. Cut into 12 pieces and serve

Nutrition Facts per serving

- Total Carbohydrates: 3,2g
- Dietary Fiber: 0,8g
- Net Total Carbohydrates: 2,5g
- Protein: 0,3g
- Total Fat: 18g
- Calories: 169

Raspberries contain antioxidants such as Vitamin C, quercetin and Gallic acid which help to prevent circulatory disease and age-related decline. They are also high in ellagic acid which has been shown to have anti-inflammatory properties.

Peanut Butter Fudge

Enough to Serve: 12

Cooking Times: 15 minutes

Ingredients

- 1 cup all natural creamy peanut butter
- 1 cup coconut oil
- 1/4 cup unsweetened vanilla almond milk
- a pinch of coarse sea salt
- 1 tsp vanilla extract
- 2 tsp liquid Stevia (optional)

Preparation Steps:

1. In a microwave safe bowl, soften the peanut butter and coconut oil together. (About 1 minute on med-low heat.)
2. Combine the softened peanut butter and coconut oil with the remaining ingredients into a blender or food processor.
3. Blend until thoroughly combined.
4. Pour into a 9X4" loaf pan that has been lined with parchment paper.
5. Refrigerate until set. About 2 hours.

Nutrition Facts per serving

- Total Carbohydrates: 4,25g
- Dietary Fiber: 1,3g
- Net Total Carbohydrates: 2g
- Protein: 5,4g
- Total Fat: 29g
- Calories: 284

IMPORTANT INGREDIENT TIP:

Coconut oil has a multitude of health benefits including improving glucose tolerance and decreasing risk of cardiovascular disease.

IMPORTANT INGREDIENT TIP:

Rich and Creamy Fat Bomb Ice Cream

Enough to Serve: 8

Ingredients

- 4 whole pastured eggs
- 4 yolks from pastured eggs
- 1/2 cup melted cocoa butter
- 1/4 cup melted coconut oil
- 15-20 drops Liquid Stevia
- 1/2 cup cocoa powder
- 1 cup MCT oil
- 2 tsp pure vanilla extract
- 8-10 ice cubes

Preparation Steps:

1. Add all ingredients but the ice cubes into the jug of your high speed blender. Blend on high for 2 minutes, until creamy.

2. While the blender is running, remove the top portion of the lid and drop in 1 ice cube at a time, allowing the blender to run about 10 seconds between each ice cube.

3. Once all of the ice has been added, pour the cold mixture into a 9×5" loaf pan and place in the freezer. Set the timer for 30 minutes before taking out to stir. Repeat this process for 2-3 hours, until desired consistency is met.

4. Serve immediately. Top with chopped nuts or shaved dark chocolate, if desired.

5. Store covered in the freezer for up to a week.

Nutrition Facts per serving

- Total Carbohydrates: 2,21g
- Dietary Fiber: 1,20g
- Net Total Carbohydrates: 0,2g

- Protein: 0,7g

- Total Fat: 25,4g

- Calories: 230

MCTs are medium-chain triglycerides, a form of saturated fatty acid that has numerous health benefits, ranging from improved cognitive function to better weight management. Coconut oil contains about 65% MCTs, but pure MCT oil can be found at many health food stores and online retailers.

One last thing

If you enjoyed this book or find it useful, I'd be very grateful if you would post short review on Amazon, your support really does make a difference and I read all of the reviews personally so I can get your feedback and make that book even better.

If you would like to give a review, then all you need to do is click the reviewer link on this book's page on Amazon here

Thanks again for your support.

www.ingramcontent.com/pod-product-compliance
Lightning Source LLC
Chambersburg PA
CBHW051758250726
48659CB00001B/496